THE LITTLE BLACK BOOK OF DENTAL WHITENING

THE LITTLE BLACK BOOK OF DENTAL WHITENING

Hendrik B. Lai

Mosen Fofel Publishing, Sheboygan, WI

COPYRIGHT

Published by Mosen Fofel Publishing, Sheboygan, WI, USA.

ISBN 978-0-6481100-2-6

ABOUT THE AUTHOR

Dr. Hendrik B. Lai is an entrepreneur, practicing dental surgeon, business consultant and an Adjunct Senior Lecturer at the College of Medicine and Dentistry at James Cook University. He is a founder and principal consultant at Schleining, Eldred, Lai and Company and serves as a Director of American Pacific Investments. Hendrik is also author of business and wellbeing books including *Teethonomics* and *Healing the Healer*.

Hendrik is passionate about helping professionals build successful businesses and has been featured by dozens of media outlets including the Sydney Morning Herald, ABC, Channel Seven, Channel TEN and Australia Network News. He has spoken extensively on health economics, strategy and health care access issues.

Hendrik and his wife, Sylvia, are the proud parents of Helena and Ethan and reside in Sheboygan County, Wisconsin.

DISCLAIMER

CONTENTS

Introduction

Thanks in large part to the popularity of television shows like The Swan and Extreme Makeover, we have seen public interest in cosmetic and esthetic procedures increase significantly over the past couple of decades. This public interest extends to include a number of appearance enhancing dental procedures.

Introduction

As you are likely aware, there is a range of dental procedures that can improve the color of teeth such as dental crowns, dental veneers and dental bonding. However, for the purposes of this book, we will limit our discussion to the improvement of tooth color achieved through chemical means.

So why is dental whitening so popular? What I've found is that there are many subtle reasons underpinning the popularity of dental whitening, but perhaps the two most important are: having a healthier appearance and increased self-confidence. Studies looking into interpersonal communications found that a whiter, more youthful smile conveys a message of health to others. Recent research tells us that a person's smile is the most memorable feature when meeting someone.

Introduction

A study conducted by the University of Manchester's School of Dentistry found a link between changes in oral health, such as how someone perceives their own smile, and their quality of life. The researchers reported that following treatment to improve the appearance of their smiles, patients reported an increase in self-confidence and overall happiness. Now, I'd ask you "who doesn't want to live a happier life?"

Armed with an understanding of the key reasons why people undertake dental whitening, we will now briefly explore the current market for the procedure and just how popular dental whitening currently is.

If we consider the United Kingdom alone, consumer surveys provide an estimate that more than 100,000 people tried tooth whitening procedures in just the past year.

Introduction

And it's not just end consumers reporting this level of popularity. Survey results of dental professionals reveal that nearly nine out of ten orthodontists had patients that requested dental whitening. The message that these surveys convey is clear: people are not only interested in dental whitening procedures, they are also actively asking for it.

From a business perspective, what we find when we delve into the numbers is that this high level of interest and popularity translates into big money. Data from the American Academy of Cosmetic Dentistry places the total annual revenue of the dental whitening industry in the order of $11 billion. Annual spending on non-prescription tooth whitening products is estimated to be around $1.4 billion - about the same as the total Gross Domestic

Introduction

Product of the Seychelles.

This means that the addition of dental whitening procedures to your dental or cosmetic practice makes good business sense. These procedures have the potential to create significant top line revenue and provide a funnel to promote complementary aesthetic and cosmetic procedures.

Despite the general popularity of the procedure, what I have found in my experience in teaching and clinical practice is that there is generally a poor understanding of dental whitening procedures. I have also found that the subject of dental whitening is an area that not a lot of time is given over to covering in dental schools. This is unsurprising given the vast amount of knowledge that needs to be imparted in dental schools, leaving elective treatments like dental whitening to be somewhat glossed over.

I have written this book to provide you with the foundations necessary to successfully implement dental whitening into your practice. This book is not intended as a replacement for adequate training in dental whitening techniques. It goes without saying that you should check the conditions of your licensure and indemnity insurance to make sure you are compliant with applicable legislation and statutes before undertaking any new procedures.

A Brief History of Dental Whitening

Patient: "Doctor, I have yellow teeth. What should I do?"

Dentist: "Wear a brown tie."

I first heard this joke many years ago when I was still in dental school. At that time we could get away with giving this flippant advice. However, the dawn of the information age has made health and wellness information more accessible to the public than ever before. Any patient concern, cosmetic or otherwise, needs to be addressed in a manner that is efficient, effective and emotionally sensitive.

Historically, the dental profession has been quite responsive to demands from patients for new and different treatment options for a variety of concerns. Treatments for improving tooth color have a long history in dentistry.

Dental bleaching is known to have been performed as early as 1848, with one of the first dental whitening procedures being described by Dwinelle in 1850. This non-vital dental whitening procedure attempted to whiten intrinsic, or internal staining often caused by damage to or the death of the nerve or blood supply to the tooth, by using chloride of lime. Chloride of lime is now commonly used to sanitize public swimming pools and as a disinfectant.

Since then, a number of different agents have been used for non-vital dental whitening procedures, including some highly toxic materials such as Labarraque's solution also known as sodium hypochlorite or more commonly liquid bleach. Also used was potassium cyanide, a chemical commonly used in electroplating, and well known for its toxicity to humans in very small quantities (as little as 200mg being a lethal dose).

A Brief History of Dental Whitening

The whitening of living, or vital, teeth goes as far back as 1892, where there are vague descriptions of tooth whitening involving a solution of 25% hydrogen peroxide and 75% ether, called Pyrozone. In 1968, Latimer described a process using oxalic acid as a whitening agent. Oxalic acid is the active ingredient in some modern abrasive cleansers including Bar Keeper's Friend and many cleansers designed to remove rust.

During this same period, dental whitening as we would recognize it today was described by an orthodontist, Dr. Bill Klusmier, in 1968. Dr Klusmier advocated the use of an oral antiseptic agent containing 10% carbamide peroxide which was delivered by specially made custom fitted mouth trays.

A Brief History of Dental Whitening

Modern commercial dental whitening commenced in the late 1980s. Prior to this time, products used to whiten teeth were primarily designed for other applications; the whitening effect was merely a pleasant side effect of the application of these products to teeth.

In 1989 Haywood and Heymann, published the first scientific studies conducted on dental whitening, coining the term "night guard vital bleaching" and legitimizing the practice of bleaching by introducing scientific evidence. 1989 also brought the first patent for products specifically designed for the purpose of dental whitening, and the first commercial at-home dental whitening product to become available to consumers.

A Brief History of Dental Whitening

Both vital and non-vital dental whitening techniques continue to be developed and refined. Many new commercial products have been introduced to the market, but all are broadly based on the same scientific principals as the peroxide-based whitening agent Pyrozone, used historically as far back as 1892.

Dental Staining

As mentioned earlier, the primary intent of dental whitening procedures is to improve the color of teeth. In order for the correct dental whitening procedure to be selected and undertaken, it is necessary to have at least a general understanding of the different types of color problems that can affect teeth.

This understanding will also allow you to better predict the rate and degree to which tooth color will improve, and in turn, better manage the expectations of your patients or clients.

Broadly speaking, tooth discoloration can be described as extrinsic or intrinsic staining. We will consider each of these broad categories in more detail in the coming pages.

Extrinsic Staining

Extrinsic stains, as the name implies is discoloration associated with the external surfaces of the teeth. Extrinsic stains usually result from an accumulation of chromatogenic substances on the external tooth surface. A chromatogenic substance is

14

an agent that causes the production of a color or a pigment.

There are a number of causes of extrinsic stains including:

1. Poor oral hygiene
2. Eating or drinking chromatogenic food and drink
3. The use of tobacco products

Rarely is a single specific issue responsible, and more often than not, it is a combination of these three factors that contributes to the formation of extrinsic stains.

Dental Staining

Extrinsic stains are largely confined to the dental pellicle. The dental pellicle is a very thin acellular layer (about a tenth of the thickness of a human hair) that is comprised of salivary glycoproteins and other macromolecules that sit on the external surface of the dental enamel.

This pellicle layer forms naturally and helps to protect the tooth surface from acid. The pellicle occurs when salivary proteins are selectively attached to the enamel surface through calcium bridges. The glycoproteins that comprise the pellicle contain proteins rich in the amino acid proline that facilitate the adhesion of bacteria allowing for the formation of dental biofilm, more commonly known as plaque.

Dental Staining

Extrinsic stains typically come about through one of two mechanisms. The first and most widely encountered is the retention of exogenous (originating from outside the body) chromophores in the dental pellicle.

We can think of a chromophore as the part of a molecule that is responsible for its color. For the purposes of our discussion about dental whitening, we can consider a chromophore to be an atom or a molecule responsible for the color of a compound. An example of a commonly encountered chromophore is the polyphenol called tannin. Tannins are found in chocolate, red wine and tea where they are largely responsible for the brown staining often seen in teacups.

Dental Staining

Exogenous chromophores are thought to form the initial attachment and retention to the dental pellicle through the interaction of chromogens with the dental pellicle via hydrogen bridges.

The second mechanism of extrinsic stain formation is discoloration caused by the Maillard reaction. If you are a cook, you may already be familiar with the Maillard reaction. This reaction is what gives seared steaks their distinctive taste and color. More specifically, the Maillard reaction is a form of non-enzymatic browning that is caused by the chemical reaction between amino acids and reducing sugars.

A reducing sugar is any sugar that is capable of acting as a reducing agent. You may recall that a reducing agent is one that donates an electron in a Reduction-

Dental Staining

Oxidation (Redox) reaction. The most common dietary sugars including galactose, fructose and glucose are all reducing sugars, so it makes sense that we might encounter this reaction in the oral cavity.

The important practical implication is that because extrinsic stains are largely confined to the dental pellicle most discoloration caused by extrinsic staining can be removed by routine professional and home based prophylactic procedures. These procedures include thorough home based tooth brushing and professional "scale and clean" procedures. With this in mind, extrinsic stains also tend to be highly responsive to chemically based dental whitening procedures.

Intrinsic Staining

As you can no doubt imagine, intrinsic stains are largely the opposite of extrinsic stains. Intrinsic stains are not confined to the external enamel surface of teeth, but rather these stains arise from a discoloration of the deeper internal dental tissue or from defects in the structure of the dental enamel.

So what causes intrinsic staining? Theoretically, the presence of any chromogenic material within the internal structure of tooth can cause internal stains. However, from a practical clinical perspective there are a number of commonly encountered causes of internal staining.

Dental Staining

Aging. Aging is arguably the most commonly encountered cause of intrinsic discoloration, perhaps because we all go through the aging process. In age related intrinsic staining, the dental tissue that underlies the dental enamel, known as dentine tends to darken as a result of the formation and deposition of secondary or tertiary dentine.

Dentine is a relatively soft calcified tissue (with a Mohs hardness of 3, which for comparison is around the same as copper) that supports the harder and more brittle dental enamel. It is comprised of approximately 70% inorganic material (largely hydroxyapatite and amorphous calcium phosphate), 20% organic material (mostly collagen with a small amount of protein known as ground substance), with the remaining 10% being water.

Dental Staining

Dentine tends to be quite porous with a characteristic yellow hue. It is this yellowness that is a common source of concern for patients about the color of their teeth. The deposited secondary or tertiary dentine is usually darker and more opaque than the original or primary dentine. Secondary dentine is structurally similar to primary dentine and is usually deposited over the life of the tooth primarily around the pulp chamber.

On the other hand, tertiary dentine tends to have a somewhat higher mineral content than primary dentine and is usually deposited in the tooth in response to a stimulus such as dental caries (dental decay).

The deposition of secondary or tertiary dentine when combined with the thinning of the overlying lighter colored and naturally translucent dental enamel due to dental wear (abrasion, attrition or erosion) results in visibly darker teeth.

Dental fluorosis may also cause internal staining. Excessive intake of fluoride during tooth formation such as through excessive ingestion of fluoride toothpaste or improper use of fluoride supplements can result in a condition known as dental fluorosis.

Dental fluorosis can be classified on a scale ranging from very mild (the most commonly encountered variety) to severe.

In cases of very mild dental fluorosis, small irregular paper white opaque areas can be seen to cover up to 25% of the tooth. In severe cases of dental fluorosis all of the enamel surfaces are affected with widespread brown staining, pitting and a "corroded" appearance.

It is believed that the discoloration associated with dental fluorosis is due to the hypomineralized enamel associated with fluorosis having altered optical properties resulting in affected dental enamel appearing opaque and less lustrous vis-à-vis unaffected dental enamel.

Internal staining caused by *drug ingestion*, particularly tetracycline antibiotics ingestion. Tetracyclines are a broad family of antibiotics, which are derivatives of polycyclic naphthacene carboxamide and are used to treat a very broad range of conditions including acne, urinary tract infections and some sexually transmitted diseases.

If tetracycline antibiotics are ingested during the development of teeth, the medication may be incorporated into the dentine through calcium chelation causing the formation of tetracycline-calcium-orthophosphate.

On exposure to ultraviolet light, such as ambient sunlight, the tetracycline-calcium-orthophosphate discolors causing varying degrees of discoloration ranging from light yellow (caused by oxytetracycline) to gray-brown (caused by chlortetracycline).

While tetracycline staining most commonly originates in childhood when the teeth are forming, there are some reports that adults using tetracyclines chronically have acquired tetracycline staining even after complete tooth development.

Discoloration of the teeth is associated with certain *inherited conditions*, especially amelogenesis imperfecta and dentinogenesis imperfecta. These conditions are caused by genetic mutations that affect the normal formation of the dental enamel in the case of amelogenesis imperfecta and the dentine in the case of dentinogenesis imperfecta. In both conditions a grey, brown or yellow discoloration of the teeth can result.

Discoloration due to *porphyria*. Porphyria is an inherited condition that affects the level of heme produced resulting in an increase in the levels of substances involved in making heme. In erythropoetic porphyria, teeth are discolored brown.

Dental Staining

Hyperbilirubinemia may also cause internal tooth staining. Hyperbilirubinemia is a condition that results from higher than normal levels of bilirubin in the blood. Bilirubin is a yellow compound that forms naturally when red blood cells break down. It is responsible for the yellowish discoloration associated with bruising and jaundice.

Newborns suffering from neonatal hyperbilirubinemia where the liver cannot properly process bilirubin often resulting in jaundice are at particular risk of developing hyperbilirubinemia associated intrinsic staining.

Trauma to the teeth that interrupts the blood supply to the tooth can result in discoloration due to decomposition of blood in the tooth. Disruption to the venous microcirculation in the tooth can result in a red discoloration which transitions to a bluish-brown discoloration.

Dental trauma resulting in *pulpal necrosis* (death of the dental pulp) can result in discoloration due to the breakdown of the pulpal tissue and blood resulting in breakdown pigments being incorporated into the dentine of the tooth.

Dental caries (dental decay) is caused by the action of cariogenic (decay causing) bacteria on fermentable carbohydrates causing the production of acidic metabolites, particularly lactic acid. This acid causes demineralization of the dental tissue.

Dental Staining

Incipient carious lesions, confined to the enamel of the tooth, may present with an opaque, matt white discoloration on the tooth. As dental caries progresses, and the dentine of the tooth becomes affected, discoloration of the tooth may occur due to the process of deposition of tertiary dentine.

Previous dental treatment may cause internal discoloration to teeth. Some dental restorations, particularly metallic restorations such as dental amalgam, may release metallic components or corrosion products that can cause discoloration in the teeth.

Furthermore, *endodontic treatment* (root canal treatment) can induce internal staining, although the mechanism of tooth discoloration due to root canal treatment is not well understood. However, it is believed that endodontic associated discoloration can be caused by incomplete debridement of pulpal tissue, certain endodontic treatment materials, especially those used to fill the root canal system at the end of endodontic therapy such as gutta percha and some endodontic sealants.

There is also some evidence to suggest that incorporation of dietary chromagens in dentinal tubules due to an absence of pulp pressure in the dentinal tubules following extirpation (removal) of the dental pulp may cause internal staining.

The practical implication here is that by their nature, intrinsic stains cannot be removed by regular prophylactic procedures as these procedures only affect the external surface of the tooth. However, intrinsic stains do respond to dental whitening agents that can penetrate the dental enamel and dentine.

Yellow age related intrinsic staining tends to respond the most rapidly to chemical dental whitening procedures. Brownish intrinsic staining is moderately responsive to dental whitening. Blue-gray tetracycline associated intrinsic stains tend to be the slowest to respond to chemical dental whitening procedures.

Dental Whitening Procedures

Now that we know about the different types of staining and some of the specific practical implications that may arise, we'll explore the different types of dental whitening procedures currently in use.

Dental Whitening Procedures

As you will recall, extrinsic stains can often be successfully removed by routine prophylactic procedures such as professional dental scaling and cleaning and good home based oral hygiene. This being the case, I will be directing most of our discussion towards improving discoloration due to intrinsic staining, although the same principles may largely be applied to improving extrinsic stains.

Broadly speaking, dental whitening can be categorized into either vital tooth whitening or non-vital tooth whitening. The underlying principles used in vital and non-vital tooth whitening procedures are similar, with the main distinction being whether the pulp of the tooth is alive and viable (as in a healthy tooth); or is no longer alive or is non-viable (as in a tooth with a necrotic pulp or a tooth which has undergone endodontic treatment).

Dental Whitening Procedures

In the next pages we will explore vital and non-vital tooth whitening procedures in more detail.

Non-Vital Tooth Whitening

Non-vital tooth whitening procedures are performed on teeth where the pulp has been removed, most commonly following endodontic treatment (root canal therapy) on the tooth. Non-vital tooth whitening is usually performed on anterior (front) teeth and it is relatively uncommon for the procedure to be performed on the posterior (back) teeth, although generally there is no contraindication to doing so.

You may recall from the earlier chapter on the history of tooth whitening that the first tooth whitening procedure described was a non-vital tooth whitening procedure using chloride of lime. Since then, the techniques used in non-vital whitening procedures have been refined with a number of techniques being in use today.

Walking Bleach Technique

The classic walking bleach technique was first described by Spasser in 1961. It involves placing a slurry of water and sodium perborate into the pulp chamber of the tooth to be whitened and sealing the slurry into the tooth with a temporary filling material.

The exhausted whitening agent is then removed from the tooth and if necessary fresh whitening agent can be placed into the pulp chamber with the process being repeated until the desired color is achieved.

This technique is considered to be the gold standard against which other non-vital whitening techniques are measured.

Modified Walking Bleach Technique

In 1967 Nutting and Poe described this technique that is a modification of the Walking Bleach Technique described above. This non-vital whitening procedure substitutes the sodium perborate and water slurry for a mixture of 30% hydrogen peroxide and sodium perborate.

In a similar manner to the Walking Bleach Technique, the slurry of hydrogen peroxide and sodium perborate is sealed into the pulp chamber of the tooth to be whitened for approximately a week. Studies have shown that there is little difference in tooth whitening effectiveness between the Walking Bleach and Modified Walking Bleach Techniques.

Internal Non-Vital Power Bleaching

In this technique a 30-35% hydrogen peroxide gel is placed into the pulp chamber of the tooth to be whitened. This hydrogen peroxide gel is then activated by light or heat, with a temperature of between 50-60°C being achieved and maintained for five minutes.

Dental Whitening Procedures

The tooth is allowed to cool back to normal body temperature (this takes approximately five minutes) and the exhausted whitening gel is washed from the pulp chamber. Current research suggests that the dramatic whitening results achieved by the internal non-vital power bleaching technique are largely short-term in nature and can be attributed to dehydration of the tooth caused by the heating process.

Studies looking into the effectiveness of this technique have concluded that the results achieved by non-vital power whitening are no better than the Walking Bleach Technique.

Dental Whitening Procedures

I suggest that you approach the Non-Vital Power Bleaching technique with caution, as there is evidence to suggest that this technique may result in root resorption due to the increased temperature within the pulp cavity.

Due to the short-lived nature of the results of this whitening technique, I suggest that this technique should be combined with the Walking Bleach Technique in order to achieve acceptable long-term results.

Inside/Outside Bleaching Technique

This technique was first described in 1997 by Settembrini et al. As the name implies, in this technique the whitening agent is applied simultaneously to both the internal and external surfaces of the tooth.

Dental Whitening Procedures

In this technique the pulp chamber access remains open for the duration of the treatment. A low concentration of whitening agent (typically 10% carbamide peroxide) is delivered to the tooth by means of a specially designed home whitening tray. This home whitening tray is designed in such a way that the whitening agent is excluded contact with the adjacent teeth.

The patient wears the whitening tray containing the whitening agent overnight. I have found that the Inside/Outside Bleaching Technique is best suited where simultaneous whitening of non-vital and vital teeth is possible and required.

Studies have concluded that after six months, this technique yields comparable results to the Walking Bleach Technique. A major disadvantage of the Inside/Outside Bleaching Technique is the lack of bacterial control because the pulp chamber access remains unsealed.

This potentially allows access of bacteria and exogenous chromagens into the tooth and this may ultimately compromise the whitening result and the longer-term success of the root canal therapy.

Vital Tooth Whitening

Vital tooth whitening is performed on teeth where the teeth are viable and the pulp remains vital. Because the pulp of the tooth is still capable of responding to stimuli, the potential for sensitivity due to the whitening process and resultant patient discomfort exists. Broadly speaking there are three available methods for the whitening of vital teeth.

In-Office Tooth Whitening

This technique is performed in the dental surgery by a dentist or a suitably qualified and trained dental auxiliary such as an oral health therapist or dental hygienist on the prescription of, and under the supervision of a dentist or where permitted by law a licensed aesthetician in their professional rooms.

In-office dental whitening techniques typically utilize a high concentration of tooth whitening agent most often employing a 25-40% hydrogen peroxide gel.

It is worth noting that many jurisdictions prohibit the supply of tooth whitening agents containing more than 6% hydrogen peroxide (or an equivalent amount of oxygen releasing product) to non-professional personnel (i.e. non-dentists).

In the in-office whitening procedure, the oral soft tissues including the gums are first protected with a suitable barrier such as rubber dam or liquid dam barrier. The whitening agent is then applied to the teeth. Although not strictly required, I recommend prophylactic cleaning of the teeth to be whitened in order to remove extrinsic staining and the dental pellicle prior to application of the whitening agent.

Dental Whitening Procedures

Some manufacturers recommend that the whitening agent should be "activated" by heat or light to enhance the whitening effect. Activation of the whitening agent is typically accomplished by halogen curing lights, plasma arc lamps, Xenon-halogen lights, diode lasers or metal halide lamps.

Most studies have concluded that there is little difference in efficacy between activated and non-activated in-office tooth whitening. However, there is some limited evidence to suggest that activation of the whitening agent with a halogen lamp may result in improved efficacy, although it is likely this effect is temporary and is due largely to the dehydration of the tooth.

There is evidence that suggests activated in-office whitening techniques may have adverse effects on the dental pulpal tissue due to increases in dental pulpal temperatures beyond the critical value of 5.5 degrees Celsius. Increases in the dental pulp temperature beyond this range can result in irreversible pulpitis or dental pulp necrosis.

At-home or Dentist-supervised Night guard Vital Bleaching (NGVB)

This technique is arguably the most widely performed dental whitening procedure and is the benchmark against which other tooth whitening procedures are measured.

Unlike the in-office tooth-whitening procedure described previously, the night guard vital bleaching technique (NGVB) is carried out by the patient under the supervision and guidance of a dentist. This supervision should include an appropriate review at dental recall appointments. Some jurisdictions may also allow non-dental personnel to provide this treatment, but you should check with your relevant local authority or licensing body.

The NGVB involves the use of a low concentration of the whitening agent, typically 10-20% carbamide peroxide, although hydrogen peroxide based formulations are also available. The whitening agent is delivered to the tooth surface by a custom fabricated night guard or dental whitening tray. For comparison, a 10-20% concentration of carbamide peroxide yields oxygen release equivalent to 3.5-6.5% of hydrogen peroxide.

Dental Whitening Procedures

Current recommendations provide that formulations containing 10% carbamide peroxide be used for eight hours per day. These lower concentration carbamide peroxide agents are hence suitable for overnight use. Higher concentrations of carbamide peroxide, typically in the 15-20% range should be limited to 4 hours per day. As such these should be reserved for daytime use.

There is good research evidence that suggests that two weeks of dentist supervised overnight NGVB with a 10% carbamide peroxide gel yields the greatest change in tooth color. With this in mind, the research suggests that all vital whitening systems result in a clinically detectable improvement in tooth color.

Dental Whitening Procedures

The design of dental whitening trays used in NGVB is a source of contention in the dental profession and there are a number of different dental tray designs currently in use with the NGVB technique. Broadly speaking, the most common permutations of dental trays are:

- Single layer or laminate trays
- With or without reservoir
- Scalloped or straight gingival margins
- With or without an incisal edge vent

The available research quite clearly shows that there is no difference in whitening efficacy between a dental whitening tray with a reservoir and one without, with the use of a reservoir for the whitening agent being the preference of the dentist or dental technician fabricating the dental tray.

Straight tray margins can result in excess whitening agent being held against the oral soft tissue with the possibility of causing chemical burns. Scalloping of the gingival margins of the dental tray provides a route for the venting of excess whitening material.

However, in this case excess whitening agent will be vented onto the oral soft tissues. This may also cause soft tissue irritation. Patients should be encouraged to use the smallest possible quantity of whitening agent to mitigate this risk.

Dental Whitening Procedures

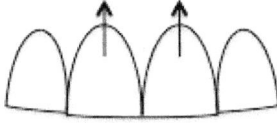

Scalloped margins can cause the whitening agent to
vent towards the oral soft tissue

Should a vented design be desired, an
incisal vent allows any excess whitening
agent to be vented away from the oral soft
tissues minimizing the risk of soft tissue
irritation.

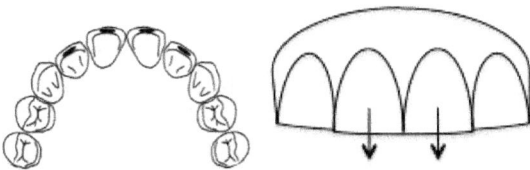

Incisal edge perforations allows venting of the
whitening agent away from the oral soft tissue

Dental Whitening Procedures

The use of a laminate dental tray design results in a more rigid dental tray that resists flexion away from the tooth surface, resulting in improved apposition of the dental tray to the tooth surface, in turn minimizing the escape of the whitening agent. The down side is that a laminate tray will tend to be somewhat thicker than a single layer tray, with the possibility of compromising patient comfort during wear.

In practice, there does not seem to be a significant difference in clinical efficacy between the different dental tray designs, with the available research showing that each permutation of tray design described above is effective in dental whitening.

I personally prefer to employ a laminate dental tray design with an incisal vent and a straight gingival margin. I do not typically use a reservoir for dental whitening tray designs used in the NGVB technique.

Once the optimal level of tooth whitening has been achieved, maintenance of the color may be performed using NGVB. You should note that the optimal level of tooth whitening is not necessarily the same as the desired level of tooth whitening. It is important to set realistic and achievable expectations with patients in order to avoid disappointment.

The current recommended frequency for "top-up" whitening is not more than once per six months, with one "top-up" day/night for every three initial whitening day/nights being a good guideline. For example, if a patient whitened their teeth for 12 nights initially, a 4-night top-up in 6-12 months would be appropriate.

Dental Whitening Procedures

High concentration whitening agent formulations (35% hydrogen peroxide) are also available. These formulations are delivered by custom fabricated dental trays in the dental office under professional supervision. This is necessary due to the risk of damage to the oral soft tissue. These formulations are typically followed by the application of at-home whitening gels containing 10-20% carbamide peroxide delivered by a custom fabricated dental tray as described above.

The rationale for this method is that applying the high concentration of whitening agent in office initiates a more rapid whitening process, although there is an increased risk of adverse side effects.

Evidence suggests that six months post whitening, there is no difference in tooth color when using a high concentration in-office tray delivered agent followed by at-home applications of carbamide peroxide and only using an at-home whitening technique.

Over-the-Counter (OTC) Dental Whitening

Over-the-Counter (OTC) dental whitening products represent the fastest growing sector of the dental market. This market segment has increased in popularity over the past number of years largely due to the low entry cost and ready availability of these products. These products are readily available for purchase without prescription in supermarkets and pharmacies.

Dental Whitening Procedures

OTC dental whitening products are composed of a low concentration of the whitening agent, typically 1-6% hydrogen peroxide and are delivered by preloaded dental trays, strips, toothpastes or paint-on solutions. Typically the products are applied twice per day for two weeks.

The effectiveness of modern OTC dental whitening products, particularly strip delivered products, compare very favorably with the benchmark professional NGVB technique. Some research even suggests superior whitening results and lower rates of sensitivity with OTC dental whitening strips versus NGVB dental whitening techniques.

OTC dental whitening products should be approached with caution as not all OTC dental whitening products have been assessed for safety and efficacy.

How Does Tooth Whitening Work?

Despite the growing popularity of dental whitening, we do not really have a good understanding of how tooth whitening with hydrogen and carbamide peroxide works. In this section, we will explore the "mechanism of action" of dental whitening using contemporary and relevant information.

How Does Tooth Whitening Work?

At its core dental whitening is fundamentally a reduction-oxidation (Redox) reaction. Hydrogen peroxide is a strong oxidizing agent that causes the molecules it reacts with to lose electrons. The hydrogen peroxide simultaneously undergoes a reduction process as it gains these electrons.

Our current understanding of tooth whitening with hydrogen peroxide or carbamide peroxide is that whitening occurs due to the presence of unstable free radicals including perhydroxyl anions, superoxide anions and hydroxyl radicals.

These free radicals can be formed by dissociation of hydrogen peroxide and hemolytic cleavage of the chemical bonds in hydrogen peroxide. There is some evidence to suggest that the formation of hydroxyl ions from hydrogen peroxide can be increased by the application of light or laser energy to the hydrogen peroxide whitening agent, enhancing the Redox reaction.

As the hydrogen peroxide whitening agent diffuses into the tooth, the free radicals formed from the dissociation of hydrogen peroxide causes the tooth whitening process by breaking down the double bonds of organic chromophore molecules.

These organic chromophores are present in the spaces between the inorganic components of tooth enamel. Broadly speaking, an organic molecule is a molecule that contains carbon atoms either in a long chain or in a ring.

How Does Tooth Whitening Work?

The complex organic molecules that are involved in dental discoloration typically possess multiple conjugated bonds. The conjugated bonds in these molecules exist in alternating double bond - single bond - double bond, etc., arrangements.

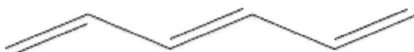

Example of a conjugated double bond arrangement

The breakdown of the double bonds in the organic chromophore molecules results in shorter chained, unconjugated molecules. This shortening of the length of the carbon chains and reduction in conjugation in turn alters the absorption spectrum of chromophore molecules effectively making the chromophores appear clear or white in the visible light spectrum

How Does Tooth Whitening Work?

The mechanism of action of tooth whitening is slightly different in tetracycline-stained teeth. In this case, the discoloration is due to photo-oxidation of organic tetracycline molecules as they are exposed to ultraviolet light.

When the whitening agent is applied to a tetracycline stained tooth, the whitening occurs through the chemical degradation of the unsaturated quinone derivative structures found in tetracycline. Quinones and quinone derivatives are a class of cyclic organic compounds that are used in industry to produce blue color dyes amongst other industrial and medicinal uses.

Effects of Dental Whitening on Oral Tissues

We now know how our whitening agent affects the chromophores that the dental whitening process is intended to act upon; however it is near impossible to target the molecules that cause dental discoloration without affecting the surrounding soft and hard tissues. In this chapter, we will explore the effects of dental whitening on the oral tissues.

As strong oxidizing agents, hydrogen peroxide and carbamide peroxide have the potential to produce irritation in the oral soft tissue such as the gingiva and oral mucosa. At higher concentrations, typically above 30% hydrogen peroxide, these agents can produce soft-tissue chemical burns, causing blanching and sloughing of the affected soft tissue.

Generally speaking irritation and chemical burns to the oral soft tissues caused by exposure to hydrogen peroxide are reversible and does not have significant longer-term consequences.

Effects of Dental Whitening on Oral Tissues

The application of a moisturizing ointment or an ointment containing an anti-oxidant such as Vitamin E to the affected area scavenges free radicals and halts the oxidation process, quickly returning normal color to affected soft tissue.

Applying an appropriate protective barrier to the oral soft tissue prior to applying high concentration whitening agents will help to minimize soft tissue irritation and chemical burns.

At lower concentrations of hydrogen peroxide or carbamide peroxide mild soft tissue irritation may be encountered. In these cases, the irritation is typically self-limiting due to the presence of endogenous peroxidases and catalases that break down peroxide and scavenge the free radicals.

Effects of Dental Whitening on Oral Tissues

Normal color typically returns to the affected soft tissue within 24-48 hours of suspending the whitening treatment. In cases of mild soft tissue irritation, a moisturizing ointment may be applied in the same manner as described above.

Despite its long and widespread use, there remain a number of questions and concerns about the effects of dental whitening on the structure of the teeth. There has been significant research looking into the effects of dental whitening on tooth structure with the results being largely mixed.

Due to its proximity to the whitening agent, the main dental tissue that is affected by tooth whitening is the dental enamel. Diffusion of the whitening agent into the dental enamel causes structural changes to this tissue. While the bulk of the research has concluded that dental whitening has no significant effect on the dental enamel when used according to manufacturer direction there have been some conflicting studies.

These conflicting studies suggest that dental whitening, especially with high concentration whitening agents or low pH (very acidic) whitening agents, may alter the surface of the dental enamel making it more porous. It is likely that the increased porosity is due to demineralization of the enamel surface and degradation of the organic component of the dental enamel.

The practical significance of this is that in order to minimize enamel surface alterations, a pH neutral whitening agent containing the lowest effective concentration of hydrogen peroxide or carbamide peroxide should be used wherever possible. Indeed, studies conclude that there is no difference in tooth whitening effectiveness between a pH neutral and acidic whitening agent.

Secondary to changes in the dental enamel surface porosity, the hardness and wear resistance of the dental enamel may also be altered by dental whitening. Normal dental enamel is the hardest substance in the human body and ranks 5 on the Mohs hardness scale and has a Young's modulus (a measure of stiffness) of 83GPa. For comparison, high strength concrete has a Young's modulus of 30GPa and human bone has a Young's modulus of 14GPa.

In the research that found no changes to enamel surface porosity, no changes to hardness or wear resistance was found. Similarly, in the studies where changes to the porosity of enamel were found following tooth whitening, there was a decrease in the hardness and Young's modulus of the enamel.

According to the available research, photo-activation of dental whitening agents does not appear to have any effect on dental enamel hardness beyond the effects observed when using non-activated whitening materials, suggesting that the main effect of whitening on enamel is solely caused by the whitening agent.

Because the main effect of dental whitening is on dental enamel tissue, this is where the bulk of the research has been directed. However, there has been some research that explores the effect of dental whitening on dentine.

Effects of Dental Whitening on Oral Tissues

The research conducted into the effect of whitening on dentine seems to be less controversial with the majority of studies finding that dentine exposure to even low concentration whitening agents for short periods of time causes a reduction in the hardness and Young's modulus of dentine.

The practical significance of the research findings into the effect of tooth whitening agents on dentine is that exposed areas of dentine should be protected from exposure to the whitening agent either with a dental filling, rubber dam or similar barrier.

It goes without saying that given the lower mineral content of dentine compared to dental enamel, low pH whitening agents should be avoided in cases where there is exposed dentine or cementum (tooth root) due to gingival recession or gingival

Effects of Dental Whitening on Oral Tissues abrasion.

Dental whitening should be avoided or at least deferred in patients with open dental cavities or actively decayed teeth. These people should be directed to a dental practitioner for treatment of the decay prior to commencing dental whitening procedures.

Effects of Dental Whitening on Dental Restorations

Many people who seek dental whitening procedures will have had past dental fillings. Indeed, the average adult DMFT in Australia was over 12 during the period 2004-2006. The DMFT is an epidemiological measure of a person's decay experience and reflects the number of teeth that have current active decay, have been extracted or have been filled.

An average DMFT of 12 means that each adult will have on average 12 teeth which are either missing, decayed or filled, or some permutation of these. The practical significance is that it is quite likely that if you undertake tooth-whitening procedures, you will encounter a patient who has at least one existing dental filling.

For the most part, tooth whitening is performed on the front teeth for esthetic reasons to achieve an improvement in the color of the visible teeth, although whitening the back teeth is possible and not generally contraindicated.

Effects of Dental Whitening on Dental Restorations

Generally speaking, the types of dental restorative materials encountered in the front region of the mouth will be composite resin or glass ionomer fillings, although less often, dental amalgam fillings may be encountered in this area.

More recently, ceramic fillings including ceramic crowns have gained in popularity as a restorative option. We will briefly explore the effect of dental whitening materials on the various dental filling materials likely to be encountered.

Composite resin is perhaps the most popular dental filling material used in the front of the mouth. Although modern dental composite resin fillings are quite robust and durable the research suggests that there is a significant increase in the porosity and the surface roughness of composite resin fillings when exposed to even low concentrations of dental whitening agents.

The increase seen in composite resin filling surface roughness is observed in both micro-filled and nano-filled composite resin fillings – these represent the two most prevalent classes of composite resin dental fillings in contemporary use. There is also some evidence to suggest that tooth whitening agents cause oxidation of the organic resin matrix of modern composite resin fillings resulting in a softening of the fillings and increasing the risk of fracture of these fillings.

It is widely advised by dental practitioners that dental whitening does not affect the color of composite resin fillings.

Effects of Dental Whitening on Dental Restorations

However a number of studies have shown that exposure of composite resin fillings to dental whitening agents does induce a color change in the restoration. Photo cured composite resin fillings typically show less color change than chemically cured composite resin fillings when exposed to dental whitening agents. This is most likely due to lower levels of the amine substances that are generally implicated in the color instability of chemically cured composite resin fillings.

The effect of tooth whitening materials on the color of dental composite resin fillings may be used for practical benefit. There has been research that concluded that dental whitening removes staining from the external surfaces of composite resin fillings more effectively than polishing and can restore the original color of the filling. It is advisable that polishing of a composite resin filling be undertaken after exposure to tooth whitening materials to counter any possible increase in roughness on the surface of the composite resin filling.

Another popular filling used in the front segment of the mouth is glass ionomer cements (GIC) and resin modified glass ionomer cements (RMGIC). GIC and to a lesser extent RMGIC fillings seem to be more profoundly affected by dental whitening agents than composite resin fillings.

Research indicates that tooth whitening agents alter the surface properties and chemistry of GIC and RMGIC fillings causing some dissolution of the surface of the fillings and this can result in "pitting" at the surface of the filling.

Similar to composite resin fillings, the hardness of GIC and RMGIC fillings was reduced when exposed to tooth whitening materials, although the effect is more pronounced with these materials. This is likely due to the process of triturating (mixing) GIC and RMGIC fillings, which can result in a number of microscopic air bubbles being present in these fillings.

Due to the significant change in hardness of GIC and RMGIC fillings and surface dissolution of the fillings, it is recommended that exposure of these fillings to dental whitening agents be avoided. This can be accomplished by applying a protective coating of a photo cured dental resin adhesive over the filling. Alternatively, exposed GIC and RMGIC fillings should be replaced following dental whitening.

Dental amalgam fillings are generally unaffected by tooth whitening materials, although where the margins of dental amalgam fillings are chipped or pitted, a green discoloration has been reported following exposure to dental whitening agents. The practical implication is that where the marginal integrity of an amalgam filling is suspect it should be replaced to minimize the formation of the green discoloration.

Ceramic restorations are typically unaffected by dental whitening materials, although there are some reports of increased surface roughness of over-glazed ceramic

Effects of Dental Whitening on Dental Restorations

fillings exposed to dental whitening agents. Auto-glazed ceramics did not exhibit any changes in surface roughness. Given the difficulty in clinically distinguishing between auto-glazed and over-glazed ceramics, it is advisable to minimize exposure of the ceramics to whitening agents where possible. If this is not possible, the ideal treatment is to remove the ceramic restoration, sandblast the affected surfaces with aluminum oxide before re-firing the ceramic restoration and re-cementing it in the mouth.

However, this ideal case is often impractical and as such I suggest that ceramic restorations be carefully examined to assess any changes to surface texture and polished using finishing grit diamond burs and a diamond polishing paste to restore the original texture if necessary.

Other Considerations for Tooth Whitening

Tooth whitening is generally accepted as a safe and effective dental procedure. Beyond an allergy to any component of the dental whitening agent to be used, there are no strict contraindications to tooth whitening.

Other Considerations for Tooth Whitening

Generally speaking, it is recommended that prior to undertaking tooth whitening treatment, a person should have a comprehensive oral examination to check for the presence of active decay, existing fillings, gum disease and para-functional habits such as bruxism.

As mentioned earlier, it is not recommended that dental whitening be performed in cases where there are open active carious lesions. Dental whitening should ideally be deferred until after the dental decay has been addressed.

Where existing fillings are present, tooth whitening candidates should be advised of the likelihood that these fillings will need to be replaced, as well as any anticipated costs associated with this. This

Other Considerations for Tooth Whitening

should be a part of your informed consent procedure for dental whitening and will help to minimize patient disappointment and mitigate risk.

The presence of para-functional habits such as bruxism and jaw joint issues may be worsened when using dental trays, particularly for overnight dental whitening procedures and when using a laminate dental tray design. Severe active bruxism may result in the perforation or deformation of the dental trays. This can allow whitening agent to escape and cause irritation to the oral soft tissue.

While there is no evidence to suggest that tooth whitening is harmful during pregnancy, tooth whitening is generally not recommended during pregnancy due to the

Other Considerations for Tooth Whitening

absence of definitive proof that the procedure is safe. While hydrogen peroxide does possess a mutagenic capacity, current research shows no evidence of carcinogenetic or teratogenetic activities in intact animal models.

There have also been reports of irritation to the mucosa of the gastrointestinal tract, including chemical burns to the hard and soft palate and throat and gastrointestinal discomfort, although these are generally attributed to improper use of dental whitening agents.

Nonetheless, in patients with pre-existing gastrointestinal complaints, including esophageal ulceration or erosion secondary to acid reflux or otherwise, clearance should sought from their attending

Other Considerations for Tooth Whitening

physician prior to commencement of the dental whitening procedure.

It goes without saying that all patients undertaking dental whitening procedures should be provided with detailed oral and written instructions and should be reviewed regularly.

Conclusion

The market is trending towards patients and the public seeking out health and wellness treatments that not only improve general wellbeing, but also have a positive cosmetic effect. Indeed in a major Australian survey, more than 20% of participants responded that they undertook non-surgical cosmetic procedures including tooth whitening within the preceding four weeks.

Conclusion

The findings of this study line up with similar research I have conducted across multiple jurisdictions that suggest nearly 25% of patients attend dental appointments with the primary goal of enhancing their appearance. This trend shows no sign of abating.

In the dental context, tooth whitening is perhaps the most conservative and cost-effective dental treatment available for improving or enhancing a person's smile. While generally regarded as very safe, as with any procedure, tooth whitening is not entirely risk-free, with only limited long-term clinical data available on the side effects of tooth whitening, although the body of knowledge continues to expand.

Conclusion

Most professional and over-the-counter tooth whitening methods utilize either carbamide peroxide or hydrogen peroxide. Although there is considerable evidence that these products whiten the teeth compared to placebo, the majority of the published scientific studies were short term and we do not have a lot of long-term evidence of the effectiveness or potential risks of tooth whitening.

While most modern techniques will whiten teeth, experience and research suggest that tooth whitening seems to be most effective when the whitening agent is placed in custom made dental trays and used overnight in order to maximize contact time between the tooth and the whitening agent.

Conclusion

Daytime dental whitening agent is the second most effective method, and realistically both techniques will yield clinically detectable improvements to tooth color.

The current available research suggests that in-office tooth whitening systems tend to result in significant improvement to the color of the teeth immediately after bleaching. However, it is not clear whether the dramatic initial results typically seen are durable, as two weeks after completing the in-office whitening treatment, there is generally no difference in tooth color between "at home" and in-office whitening procedures.

Given the potential for disturbance and damage to the dental pulp, in-office whitening should be approached with caution, especially if using an "activated" system.

Although in theory, dental whitening procedures can be carried out by anyone (where permitted by law), I recommend that tooth whitening be performed under professional supervision and only following a pre-treatment dental examination. This consultative approach to dental whitening allows for the most appropriate bleaching treatment to be chosen based on the patient's lifestyle factors, financial and oral health considerations.

Tooth whitening remains one of the most popular cosmetic dental procedures and is performed safely and effectively thousands of times every day the world over. Considering that two of the key tenets of health care are *beneficence and non-*

Conclusion

malfeasance, dental professionals and appropriately qualified and licensed cosmetic professionals are obliged to undertake and maintain adequate training to achieve safe and effective dental whitening results for patients and clients.

Given the current market expenditure on appearance enhancing dental procedures and the likely continued general interest in appearance and health more generally, with over 50% of the population in a major study self-motivated to improve their appearance, it would be a wise business decision to incorporate safe, proven and effective dental whitening offerings, that are underpinned by a sound understanding of the fundamental scientific principles of tooth whitening into your dental or cosmetic business.